Essential Oils For Kids And Babies

A Simple Guide To Aromatherapy And Using Essential Oils For Children

CORAL MILLER

Disclaimer

The information in this book is solely for informational purposes, not as a medical instruction to replace the advice of your physician or as a replacement for any treatment prescribed by your physician. The author and publisher do not take responsibility for any possible consequences from any treatment, procedure, exercise, dietary modification, action or application of medication which results from reading or following the information contained in this book.

If you are ill or suspect that you have a medical problem, we strongly encourage you to consult your medical, health, or other competent professional before adopting any of the suggestions in this book or drawing inferences from it.

This book and the author's opinions are solely for informational and educational purposes. The author specifically disclaims all responsibility for any liability, loss, or risk, personal or otherwise which is incurred as a consequence, directly or indirectly, of the use and application of any of the contents of this book.

DEDICATION

To my beautiful niece, Sharon…because you deserve the
best!

TABLE OF CONTENT

Read Other Books By Coral Miller

(Available At Popular Retailers)

Essential Oils For Your Pet: 47 Safe, Natural And Easy
Home Remedies For Fido (Aromatherapy for Dogs)

INTRODUCTION

Essential Oils, Aromatherapy And Your Kid

Essential oils are natural aromatic compounds that are found in plants. They are extracted from a large variety of aromatic herbs by steam distillation or cold- pressing. Since they are aromatic compounds of the plants from which they are extracted, they retain all the healing qualities of the mother-herb. Consequently, they are about 70 times more powerful than herbs. Although they are called "oils", they are in fact a liquid and do not feel oily at all. They are highly concentrated, extremely powerful, richly fragrant, safe and without side effects.

Essential oils are used for aromatherapy, which is the art of treating diseases with herbal essences. Aromatherapy dates back thousands of years. The ancient people discovered that aromatic compounds in essential oils have direct effect on their mental, emotional and physical health. This is holistic therapy because it not only aims for the individual's body, but for his mind and soul as well.

Babies are born with clear and beautiful skin. As they grow, they require extra care to sustain their cherubic beauty. Children's beauty tips include an extensive care that starts from skin to health. A lot of children's products such as shampoos, powders and baby wipes contain harmful chemicals. Exposing them to these harsh chemical-based beauty products and medicines is dangerous due to their tender and sensitive skin. Using natural products with essential oils will help to protect your kid's health from these harmful products. Besides good food, plenty of rest, outdoor plays and good hygiene to help kids grow and develop well, there is need to use essential oils to address their internal and external beauty needs.

These little ones must be protected from these harmful products which may have devastating health effect in the long run. Although some reputed brands have included many skin care and health products for children, choosing the right product may be difficult as manufacturers aren't always truthful about their product ingredients' and claims.

Then again, nature has its own tender way of healing and helping the body recover its energy and health. This is the only thing our kids need: a little help for their fight with an intrusive external agent. Therefore, it makes a lot of sense to use essential oil for general wellbeing.

Benefits Of Essential Oils For Kids And Babies

Essential oils provide tremendous benefits physically and emotionally. Since they come from therapeutic plants, they provide a wide range of health benefits. And since they are natural compounds without a single chemical ingredient, they are safer than commercial products, particularly when used correctly. They are affordable and also handy as they can be made quickly, easily and stored. They should be an important part of the natural remedies for every home.

Essential oils help to treat different ailments in kids and even babies. They help relieve a runny nose, get better sleep (due to their calming effect), treat some skin issues like scratches, rushes and minor bruises as well as provide relief from many ailments like fever, constipation, jaundice, hiccoughs, earaches and teething pain.

Where antibiotics cannot penetrate cell membrane, essential oils can penetrate cells to kill bacteria and viruses easily. They penetrate the skin and are quickly absorbed into the body where they fight and kill bacteria and viruses.

Essential oils can also be part of natural ingredients for baby and kids' oils, lotions, powders and wipes. As wonderful additive to natural products, they also provide these products with a unique fragrance due to their aromatic nature.

Using Essential Oils Safely For Babies And Children

Before you use essential oils for babies and children, you must exercise some measure of caution. Essential oils are extremely strong and must never be used internally on small children. Also, keep your essential oils out of the reach of babies and small children to prevent the risk of ingestion. However, if ingestion occurs, do not induce vomit but take your child immediately to the emergency ward.

Dilution of the essential oils is very important. Essential oils must always be used diluted in a carrier oil. Virgin Coconut Oil is an excellent carrier oil for babies because it is nutrient-rich but others like sunflower, almond, grape seed and apricot kernel may also be used. Other dilution material like milk, vegetable glycerin or raw honey may also be used.

Using neat (undiluted) essential oils may cause seizures or irritation to the skin. Do not use essential oils on children's face and in and around their noses. Their strong fragrance (especially the ones that contain menthol) may slow their breathing and lead to respiratory problems.

Be careful when using essential oils with babies. They may be allergic to a certain compound as you haven't discovered yet all his/her sensitivities. It is recommended that you introduce no more than an essential oil a day. After that, watch your baby's reaction. If there is an allergy problem, the effects should appear in about 30-40 minutes. The best thing you can do is to initially test a small part of the skin when applying lotions or massage oils.

When using oils with children, more isn't better. Be sure to always dilute well and use only a very small amount of oil as it goes a long way to soothe and calm. A larger quantity may lead to fussiness and agitation.

Safety Tips

Have these tips at your fingertips:

- Do not use undiluted essential oil directly on your kid's skin (burning and irritation may occur).
- If essential oils are used in bath, always disperse by using a bath gel or dilute in a water soluble carrier like vegetable glycerin or raw unfiltered honey.
- Avoid getting essential oils in eyes. If you do, flush eyes with milk.
- Do not place undiluted essential oil too close to kid's face.

- Do not use undiluted essential oil in a diffuser as the scent will be too strong for your child.
- Never ever ingest an essential oil. If ingested in error, give liquids such as cream, milk, half and half and immediately call your doctor. A few drops usually isn't life threatening but it is safer to take these precautions.
- Do not use essential oils on premature babies on account of their delicate and almost transparent skin. It is best to wait until the skin has attained more maturity.

Using Essential Oils With Children

There are different ways of using the essential oils for children such as baths, inhalations, compresses, massages and sprays. However, the easiest ways to use essential oils with babies are:

I. **Diffusion**

Diffusion involves diffusing essential oil in an oil burner or diffuser in order for it to disperse through the air and inhaled. For babies, simply add a drop of essential oil to 2 teaspoons of water and then add it to diffuser.

ii. **Massage**

To massage, create massage/body oil for your baby by combining essential oil with a carrier oil. Massage on the body so it penetrates the skin.

iii. **Inhalation**

Inhalation can be done with an inhaler, aroma lamp or with some cotton pads. If you use an inhaler, add 10 drops but only 2 drops with the cotton pads. Once the child inhales the oil from these, the therapeutic effects addresses the ailments which is usually a runny nose and congestion.

iv. **Bath**

For a calming effect and great scent, use the essential oils for the bath of children. Always dilute them in a carrier oil or in another carrier material. There is a big difference in diluting the oils for an adult and for a child. Children are more sensitive, so if you use 6 drops of essential oil to 20 ml of carrier oil for an adult, do not use more than 2-3 drops for a child.

Certain oils have repellent effects. They are effective against insect bites and in certain combinations, can keep nasty insects away from your child. You may also spray an essential oil combination or diffuse it, depending on their purpose.

Essential Oils That Are Good For Children

The correct usage of essential oil depends on the age of the baby. However, it is advisable to avoid using essential oils for babies under 3 months. This is because of their very tender skin which is also prone to allergic reactions.

For Babies 3+ Months

Use 1-2 drops of essential oil/1ounce of carrier oil. The allowed essential oils include:

Chamomile (Roman and German)
Lavender
Yarrow (Blue)
Dill

For Babies Age 6+ Months

Increase the dose to 3-5 drops of essential oil/ 1ounce of carrier oil. The allowed essential oils Include:

Sweet Orange
Tangerine
Mandarin
Sandalwood
Tea tree
Bergamot
Citronella
Geranium
Grapefruit
Neroli
Palma Rosa
Pine
Cinnamon leaf – use very small amounts (1-2 drops). It can cause skin irritation if it is not diluted properly
Cinnamon bark – only use for diffusion. It is not safe to apply on the skin as it may cause severe irritation

Be careful with Citrus essential oils as they are photo toxic. What this means is they can cause severe reactions if the skin is exposed to sunlight. Do not use this kind of essential oils when preparing a sunscreen lotion, for example. Add lavender oil instead. There are a few citrus essential oils that are not photo toxic: Mandarin, Sweet Orange, Tangerine, Lemon or Lime obtained through steam distillation process.

For Children 2+ Years

Increase the dose to 20 drops of essential oil/1ounce of carrier oil. Choose from the list below:

Lime
Lemongrass
Frankincense
Basil, Lemon
Basil, Sweet
Melissa/Lemon Balm
Tea Tree, Lemon
Ylang Ylang
Sweet Marjoram
Garlic
Clary Sage
Thyme
Verbena, Lemon
Ginger
Oregano
Patchouli
Juniper Berry

For Children 6+ Years

Here, the list gets bigger and the dose too: 30 drops of essential oil/ounce of carrier oil. Essential oils to be used:

Nutmeg
Cardamom
Laurel Leaf/Bay Laurel
Niaouli
Peppermint
Cajuput
Anise, Star
Sage, Greek/White
Anise/Aniseed
Cornmint

Children 10+ Years

Here, all the essential oils are safe for diffusion or topical use. However, be careful with the oils you haven't used before. Introduce one at a time and test it before if it is applied on the skin.

Proper care should be taken when using essential oils that contain menthol and cineole. These two compounds may cause a reflex that slows down the breathing which, in some cases, can be dangerous.

There are 3 essential oils with these constituents:

Eucalyptus
Rosemary
Peppermint (at 6+ years, peppermint is safe for children's usage)

REMEDIES FOR COMMON AILMENTS

General Guidelines For Dilution

Babies 3+ months – 1-2 drops/1ounce of carrier oil (almond, grape seed, coconut oil)

Babies 6+ months – 3-5 drops/1ounce of carrier oil
Children 2+ years – 20 drops/1ounce of carrier oil

Children 6+ years old – 30 drops/1ounce of carrier oil

Fever
For babies

Ingredients

1-2 drops Lavender essential oil

1 oz carrier oil

Directions

Combine and massage baby or child's feet, back, neck and behind the ears

Diaper Rash
For babies

Ingredients

1-2 drops Lavender essential oil
1 oz carrier oil

Dilute & apply to the irritated area

Or

Ingredients

1 drop of Lavender essential oil

1 drop of Roman Chamomile essential oil

1 drop whole milk

Directions

Add to baby's bath water.

Before bathing baby, swish around

Do not let the oils get into your baby's eyes.

Colds and Runny Nose
For young children

Ingredients

1 drop Lavender, Tea Tree, Thyme or Niaouli essential oil

1 oz carrier oil

Directions

Dilute and use for massaging baby's chest or back.

Common Cold Blend
For young children

Ingredients

2 drops Melaleuca (Tea Tree)

1 drop rose otto

1 drop lemon

2 Tbsp. vegetable oil

Directions

Combine and massage lightly on neck and chest.

Flu
For young children

Ingredients

1 drop Cypress, lemon or Melaleuca

1 Tbsp. bath gel base

Directions

Dilute in a bath or diffuse

Bruises
For young children

Ingredients

1drop Lavender

1drop Geranium

1 oz or 2tbsp carrier oil

Directions

Dilute and apply to the bruise.

Minor burns
For young children

Directions

1. Cool the skin for 10 minutes by immersing the burned skin in water.

2. If the skin isn't broken, apply 2 drops lavender essential oil directly on the burned area.

3. If the skin is broken, apply 2 drops of lavender around the burned area. Afterwards, put 5 drops of diluted lavender oil on a cold, dry cloth and then hold it over the area of the burn.

Colic Blend
For young children

<u>Ingredients</u>

1 drop of Roman Chamomile essential oil

1 drop Geranium

1 drop Lavender

2 tablespoons of almond oil

<u>Directions</u>

Blend and massage gently to the abdomen of the baby.

Cradle Cap
For babies

<u>Ingredients</u>

1 drop lemon

1 drop geranium

2 tbsp almond oil

<u>Directions</u>

Mix oils together and apply a small quantity on the head.

Crying
For babies

<u>Ingredients</u>

1-2 drops Lavender or Roman Chamomile

<u>Directions</u>

Place on hand or tissue and offer the baby to smell.

Chicken Pox
For young children

<u>Ingredients</u>

10 drops lavender

10 drops Roman Chamomile

4 oz calamine lotion

<u>Directions</u>

1. Dilute oils in calamine lotion.

2. Mix well and apply over body two times daily

Cuts And Scrapes
For young children

<u>Ingredients</u>

5 drops lavender

5 drops Malaleuca

1 drop Lavender

<u>Directions</u>

1. Dilute oils in a small bowl of warm water.

2. Use the diluted water to clean the cut.

3. Apply 1 drop lavender essential oil to band- aid

4. Use it to cover the wound.

Coughs
For babies

<u>Ingredients</u>

1 drop of Lavender

1 tbsp carrier oil

<u>Directions</u>

Combine and rub a small quantity on baby's chest and back.

Diarrhea

For babies

<u>Ingredients</u>

1 drop Roman Chamomile

1 Tbsp carrier oil

<u>Directions</u>

1. Mix together and apply2-3 drops of this mixture on the tummy.

2. Massage clockwise following the colon's natural movement

Jaundice

For babies

<u>Ingredients</u>

1 drop Geranium

1 Tbsp carrier oil

<u>Directions</u>

Mix and apply over the liver area and to the bottoms of feet.

Earache
For young children

<u>Ingredients</u>

1-2 drops lavender

1-2 drops malaleuca

<u>Directions</u>

1. Dilute these oils and apply on a cotton pad.

2. Place the pad on the surface of the ear.

3. Place piece of tape across the ear to hold the cotton in place.

4. Send Child to bed.

Hiccoughs
For babies

Diffuse diluted Mandarin essential oil

Insect Bites
For babies & young children

<u>Ingredients</u>

1-2 drop lavender oil

2 tbsp or (1 oz) fractionated coconut oil

Directions

Dilute and dot each bite

Constipation
For young children

Ingredients

1- 2 drops orange, mandarin or ginger essential oil

2tbs fractionated coconut oil

Directions

Dilute and massage a little on the feet.

Teething
For babies

Ingredients

1 drop lavender or Roman Chamomile

1 Tbsp carrier oil

Directions

Mix and use a little to massage gently along the jaw line.

Teeth grinding

Rub diluted Lavender essential oil on feet

Tummy Ache
For babies

Ingredients

1 drop Roman Chamomile

1 drop Sweet Orange

2 tbsp carrier oil

Directions

1. Mix and add 1 tsp of this mixture to warm bath water.

2. Before bathing baby, swish around and do not let the oils get into your baby's eyes.

Rashes
For young children

Ingredients

I drop Lavender

1 drop Roman Chamomile

1 teaspoon fractionated oil

Directions

Combine and apply to location

Sleeping

Use this remedy on alternative nights until your baby learns to sleep all through the night

<u>Ingredients</u>

1 drop chamomile Roman

1 drop geranium oil

1bowl boiling water

<u>Directions</u>

1. Put your baby to bed and then place on the floor beneath the cot (crib) the bowl of boiling water.

2 Add the oils to it.

3. Leave the door ajar so the aroma molecules will be contained in the baby's room.

Sunburn

For young children

<u>Ingredients</u>

5 drops lavender

1 tsp aloe Vera

Directions

Dilute oil and apply over sunburned area.

MASSAGE OILS AND LOTIONS

Homemade Baby Oil
Make your own baby oil to keep your baby happy and healthy

Suitable for babies 3+ months old

Ingredients

4 oz organic sweet almond oil
4 oz. organic olive oil

10 drops of Roman Chamomile essential oil

Directions

Combine the carrier oils and the Chamomile essential oil and mix well

Baby Balm
Use this natural balm for eczema and other skin problems. It has an incredible scent too!

Suitable for children 6+ months old

Ingredients

¼ cup cocoa butter

¼ cup Shea butter

1 Tablespoon castor oil

2 Tablespoons olive oil

10 drops Sweet Orange Essential Oil

10 drops Sandalwood Essential Oil

<u>Directions</u>

1. Melt all the ingredients in a jar over a pan half full with water or a double boiler.

2. Let cool a little bit and add the essential oils.

3. Store in a container.

4. Massage the affected area with a small amount of baby balm.

Diaper Cream

Avoid using conventional diaper creams that contain chemical ingredients. Do it yourself!

This remedy is suitable for babies 6+ months old.

<u>Ingredients</u>

1/4 cup coconut oil

1/4 cup Shea butter

2 Tablespoons of Fermented Cod Liver Oil

1 Tablespoon beeswax pastilles

2 tablespoons of zinc oxide powder

1 tablespoon of bentonite clay

5 drops Chamomile essential oil

Directions

1. Combine Shea butter, beeswax and coconut oil and melt them in a double boiler.

2. Next, let it cool for 1 minute and then add the other ingredients.

3. Mix well and distribute the zinc oxide through the mixture.

4. Place it into the store container and stir a few more times until it's cool.

5. Keep in a dark place for 3 months.

Soft Baby Oil

Avoid the petroleum based baby oils and try this vitamin rich homemade oil

Suitable for babies 6+ months old

Ingredients

1 cup olive oil/apricot kernel oil

2 tablespoons calendula flowers

2 tablespoons chamomile flowers

10 drops Roman Chamomile essential oil

Directions

1. Place the herbs in a jar and cover them with the oil. Put a lid over the jar.

2. Store in a dark place for 6-8 weeks and shake every day.

3. Remove the flowers and add the essential oil

4. Use as regular baby oil.

Homemade Lotion for Babies
Your baby will love this ultra-moisturizing lotion.

Ingredients

¼ cup coconut oil

½ cup almond or olive oil

¼ cup beeswax

1 teaspoon Vitamin E oil

5 drops Lavender essential oil

5 drops Roman Chamomile essential oil

Directions

1. Melt the coconut oil, beeswax and almond/olive oil in a double boiler or a jar placed over a sauce pan half filled with hot water.

2. Once they melt, add the Vitamin E oil and the essential oils.

3. Store in a container.

Nourishing Baby Lotion

Protect your baby's skin with this smooth lotion

Suitable for babies 3+ months old

Ingredients

3 tablespoons cocoa butter

4 tablespoons apricot oil

1 tablespoon beeswax

1/2 cup filtered water

1 tablespoon dried lavender

5 drops Roman Chamomile essential oil

Directions

1. Combine the lavender and water and bring to a boil

2. Strain the tea and place it to a blender

3. Melt the cocoa butter and the beeswax.

4. To the melted mixture, add the apricot oil.

5. Place the oil mixture in the blender too.

6. Mix until it emulsifies.

7. Store in a jar and let it cool.

Rich Baby Oil

The blend of natural oils will nourish your baby's skin

Suitable for babies 3+ months old

<u>Ingredients</u>

2 oz apricot kernel oil

2 oz sweet almond oil

2 oz grape seed oil

1 tbsp Shea butter

1 tbsp cocoa butter

1 tbsp coconut butter

Few drops vitamin E oil

2 drops Lavender essential oil

<u>Directions</u>

1. Combine all the ingredients, except for the Vitamin E oil and the essential oil, and melt them into a double boiler.

2. Let cool for a few minutes, and then add the Vitamin E and Lavender essential oil. Store them in spray bottles.

Homemade Diaper Balm
Keep your baby happy with this soothing natural balm

Suitable for babies 3+ months old

<u>Ingredients</u>

1 oz cocoa butter

1 oz beeswax

3 oz Coconut oil

2 oz avocado oil

1 teaspoon Vitamin E oil

5 drops Lavender essential oil

5 drops Roman Chamomile essential oil

<u>Directions</u>

1. Combine the Cocoa butter, beeswax, coconut oil and avocado oil and place them in a double boiler or a jar over a saucepan half full with water.

2. Heat the ingredients until they melt, stirring a few times.

3. Let cool a little bit. Add the Vitamin E oil and the essential oils.

4. Store in a container.

Baby Smooth Balm

This balm can heal cuts, burns, rashes, scrapes, chapped lips.

Suitable for babies 6+ months old

Ingredients

½ cup of extra virgin olive oil

¼ cup dried calendula petals

1/8 cup of grated beeswax

8 drops of Lavender essential oil

Directions

1. Place the calendula petals and olive oil in a small slow cooker. Set the temperature on low for 3 hours.

2. Strain the oil very slowly. Mix the oil with the beeswax in a small skillet and let it heat until the beeswax melt.

3. After it cools for a few minutes, add the essential oil. Store in a dry container.

HYGIENE AND BATH

Homemade Shampoo & Body Wash
Suitable for babies 3+ months old if using only Lavender essential oil and for babies 6+ months old if using both essential oils

Ingredients

4 oz filtered water
1 oz liquid castile soap, unscented
3 drops Sweet Orange essential oil
3 drops Lavender essential oil

Directions

Mix all the ingredients in a container.

Lavender Baby Shampoo
This homemade shampoo is distinguished through its delicate lavender smell

Suitable for babies 6+ months old

Ingredients

1 cup castile soap

4 cups distilled water

1/4 cup aloe Vera gel

2 tablespoons coconut oil

3 teaspoons guar gum

1.5 teaspoon Neo Defend

2 teaspoons citric acid

30 drops Lavender essential oil

Directions

1. Put all the ingredients, except the castile soap, in a blender and mix for about 40 sec

2. Add the castile soap

3. Place the shampoo into a container.

Baby Powder
Instead of using talc on your baby's skin, try this homemade recipe.

Suitable for babies 6+ months old

Ingredients

½ cup arrowroot powder

5 drops Roman Chamomile essential oil

Directions

Combine the ingredients and store in a container.

Chamomile Baby Shampoo

This homemade shampoo will fit perfectly to your baby's soft hair.

Suitable for babies 6+ months old.

<u>Ingredients</u>

6 oz castile soap

1 teaspoon almond oil

10 drops Roman Chamomile essential oil

<u>Directions</u>

1. Mix well all the ingredients

2. Store in a clean container.

Teething Gel

Suitable for infants 2+ years old

1 drop Clove Essential Oil

1 tablespoon glycerine or vegetable oil

<u>Directions</u>

Combine in small bottle, shaking until thoroughly blended.

Milk Bath

Milk can be used as a nourishing bath additive for babies

Suitable for babies 3+ months old.

<u>Ingredients</u>

1/2 cup cornstarch

1 cup dried milk

2 to 3 drops Lavender or Chamomile essential oils

<u>Directions</u>

1. Mix well all the ingredients.

2. Put a small amount of this mixture in the warm bath.

Homemade Baby Powder

Say no to diaper rash with this natural baby powder.

Suitable for babies 6+ months old

<u>Ingredients</u>

1/4 cup arrowroot powder

1/4 cup cornstarch

1 tbsp white clay

3 drops Sweet Orange essential oil

1 drop Geranium essential oil

2 drops Sandalwood essential oil

<u>Directions</u>

Mix the ingredients and store in a jar.

Homemade Baby Wipes

Use this all natural baby wipes for your baby's hygiene.

Suitable for babies 6+ months

<u>Ingredients</u>

1/8-1/4 cup Castile soap

2 cups lukewarm water

1/8-1/4 cup vegetable oil (almond, olive, apricot seeds, etc)

Roll of paper towels

1 plastic container that the roll will fit in

5 drops Chamomile essential oil

2 drops Tea Tree essential oil

<u>Directions</u>

1. Take the roll of paper towels and cut it in half, then remove the cardboard.

2. Mix all the ingredients in the container.

3. Put the paper roll in the container, cut side down.

4. Seal the container and turn it upside down.

5. Pull the wipes from the middle in order to use.

Baby Healing Wipes

These natural baby wipes have a comforting effect on your baby's skin

Suitable for babies 6+ months old

<u>Ingredients</u>

1/4 cup Aloe Vera gel

1 1/2 to 2 cups distilled water

2 teaspoon castile soap

1 tablespoon Calendula oil

2 to 3 drops Tea Tree oil

2 to 3 drops Lavender oil

Roll of paper towels

1 plastic container that the roll will fit in

<u>Directions</u>

1. Mix all the ingredients, except for the essential oils

2. Let the mixture sit for a few minutes, then add the essential oils

3. Take the roll of paper towels and cut it in half, then remove the cardboard.

4. Place the mixture into the container.

5. Put the paper roll in the container, cut side down.

6. Seal the container and turn it upside down.

7. Pull the wipes from the middle in order to use.

Baby Bubble Bath

Let your baby enjoy his/her bath with natural bubbles.

<u>Ingredients</u>

3/4 cup water

1 cup baby shampoo or eco-friendly liquid soap

1/2 to1 teaspoon glycerin

2 drops Chamomile essential oil

2 drops Lavender essential oil

<u>Directions</u>

Mix all the ingredients and let them sit for a while before adding the essential oils.

SUNSCREEN LOTIONS

Homemade Sunscreen

Use a homemade lotion that protects and nourishes the skin of your baby.

Suitable for babies 6+ months old

<u>Ingredients</u>

¼ cup of Shea butter

¼ cup of coconut oil

2 tablespoons beeswax granules

1/8 cup almond oil

1-2 tablespoons of zinc oxide

10 drops Lavender essential oil

<u>Directions</u>

1. Place the coconut oil, Shea butter, beeswax and almond oil in a jar.

2. Heat some water in a saucepan and put the jar inside or use a double boiler. Wait for all the ingredients to melt.

3. Next, mix in the zinc oxide and refrigerate for 10 minutes. (Always use a mask when dealing with zinc oxide. Be sure to distribute it all throughout the mixture).

4. Take it out, add the Lavender essential oil and blend all the ingredients using a hand mixer.

5. Put the sunscreen in a container and use it within 6 months. Store in a dark place.

Natural Homemade Sunscreen
Protect your baby from skin irritation with this remedy

Suitable for children 6+ months old

Ingredients

1 oz coconut oil

0.8 oz shea butter
0.1 oz Vitamin E oil

0.1 oz jojoba, sesame, or sunflower oil

1 tablespoon zinc oxide powder

10 drops Lavender/Sandalwood essential oil

Directions

1. Use a double boiler to melt the following ingredients: Shea butter, coconut oil and jojoba/sunflower/sesame oil.

2. Remove the oily mixture and let it cool.

3. Using a mask, add the vitamin E oil, essential oils and the zinc oxide and evenly distribute.

4. Move the sunscreen into a container and store in a dark place.

INSECT REPELLENTS FOR CHILDREN

Homemade Insect Repellent

Did you know that all store-bought repellents contain DEET which may not be 100% safe for your children? Protect your kids today! Make your own repellent.

Suitable for children 2+ years.

Ingredients

15 drops citronella essential oil
10 drops lemongrass essential oil

10 drops lemon essential oil

5 drops cedar essential oil

1 oz witch hazel

1 oz grape seed oil

Directions

1. Mix all the ingredients in a spray bottle

2. Make sure to shake it well before applying on skin.

Water Based Bug Spray

It and protects your child from the nasty insects.

Suitable for children 2+ years old

Ingredients

2 oz water

2 oz witch hazel/vodka/apple cider vinegar

¼ teaspoon castile soap

10 drops citronella essential oil

10 drops lemongrass essential oil

10 drops tea tree oil

5 drops cedar essential oil

5 drops lemon essential oil

Directions

1. Mix the essential oils with the witch hazel/vodka/apple cider vinegar.

2. Add the castile soap and let it still for a few minutes.

3. Shake well the mixture.

4. Add the water.

5. Place the liquid into a spray bottle.

6. Shake before use

Oil Based Bug Spray
Suitable for children 2+ years old

<u>Ingredients</u>

2 oz jojoba or olive oil

10 drops citronella essential oil

10 drops lemongrass essential oil

10 drops tea tree oil

5 drops cedar essential oil

5 drops lemon essential oil

<u>Directions</u>

Mix all the ingredients and store in spray bottle.

Patchouli Bug Spray
The blend of essential oils smells great and will keep insects away.

Suitable for children 2+ years old

<u>Ingredients</u>

4 oz witch hazel/vodka/apple cider vinegar

15 drops patchouli essential oil

10 drops geranium essential oil

15 drops cedarwood atlas or cedarwood Virginia essential oil

<u>Directions</u>

1. Mix the essential oils to the witch hazel/vodka/apple cider vinegar and let it sit for a while.

2. After that mix well and add the water.

3. Store it in a spray bottle.

4. Shake well before use.

Wonder Bug Spray
Suitable for children 2+ years old

<u>Ingredients</u>

2 oz jojoba or olive oil

13 drops geranium bourbon essential oil

13 drops patchouli essential oil

13 drops cedarwood atlas or cedarwood Virginia essential oil

<u>Directions</u>

Mix all the ingredients and store in spray bottle.

Citronella Spray

Citronella essential oil with its strong repellent effect works excellently.

Suitable for children 2+ years old.

Ingredients

2 oz water

2 oz witch hazel/vodka/apple cider vinegar

15 drops cedarwood atlas or cedarwood Virginia essential oil

15 drops citronella essential oil

10 drops geranium essential oil

Directions

1. Mix the essential oils to the witch hazel/vodka/apple cider vinegar and let it sit for a while.

2. After that mix well and add the water.

3. Store it in a spray bottle.

4. Shake well before use.

Soothing Insect Spray

Use only natural ingredients for protecting your child's skin.

Suitable for children 2+ years old.

<u>Ingredients</u>

2 oz jojoba/olive oil

15 drops cedarwood atlas or cedarwood Virginia essential oil

15 drops citronella essential oil

10 drops geranium essential oil

<u>Directions</u>

Mix all the ingredients and store in a spray bottle.

Itchy Relief Repellent

Get rid of the annoying itches with this natural repellent

Suitable for children 2+ years old.

<u>Ingredients</u>

2 oz jojoba/coconut oil

10 drops neem oil

10 drops Lavender essential oil

10 drops Lemon essential oil

10 drops Thyme essential oil

10 drops Geranium essential oil

<u>Directions</u>

Mix all the ingredients and store in a bottle.

HOUSE CLEANING

Homemade Laundry Soap

Don't let all the harsh chemicals from conventional detergents touch the skin of your baby.

Suitable for babies 3+ months old

<u>Ingredients</u>

3 tablespoons washing soda

3 tablespoons borax

2 tablespoons organic dish soap

15 drops Lavender essential oil

4 cups boiling water

<u>Directions</u>

1. Mix together: borax, washing soda, dish soap and essential oils in a large container (one gallon)

2. Pour the boiling water and stir until well combined

3. Let this mixture cool.

4. Fill the container with cold water almost to the top

Homemade Liquid Laundry Soap

The soap nuts are the most harmless washing agent ever! They are just perfect for your baby's clothes.

Suitable for babies 6+ months old.

Ingredients

1 cup soap nuts

1/2 cup vinegar (natural preservative)

4 cups water

10 drops Sweet Orange essential oil

10 drops Tangerine essential oil

Directions

1. Place the soap nuts, vinegar and water into a large pot and mix them together.

2. Bring to a boil on medium-low temperature and let them simmer for 30 minutes. The lid must be on the pot.

3. Remove the lid and let boil for 30 minutes more. Stir from time to time.

4. Let the liquid cool and add the essential oils.

5. Sore into a clean container.

Perfect Stain Remover

We all know that the babies' clothes can get very dirty but this natural stain remover will help.

Ingredients

1/4 cup liquid castile soap

1 1/2 cups water

1/4 cup liquid vegetable glycerin

5-10 drops of Lemon essential oil

Directions

1. Combine all the ingredients and mix well.

2. Store in a glass container (Lemon essential oil may have a harsh effect on plastic)

Boom Liquid Dishwasher

When you wash your child's dishes there can be detergent leftovers. It is best to use a natural dishwasher in order to protect your baby.

Ingredients

1/8 cup water

1/2 cup liquid castile soap

4 drops essential oil scent of choice

1 teaspoon vinegar

Directions

Combine all the ingredients and store into an old dishwasher container.

Homemade Toy Cleaner
A cheap way to keep your child's toys clean

Ingredients

1 cup distilled white vinegar

1 cup water

3 drops Tea Tree essential oil

Directions

Mix all the ingredients and store in spray bottle.

Homemade Surface Cleaner
Keep your house clean for the safety of your children

Ingredients

2 tablespoons white vinegar

1 1/2 cups of warm water in a measuring cup

1 teaspoon liquid castile soap

2 teaspoons rubbing alcohol

8-10 drops of Tea Tree essential oil (for its antibacterial effect)

1 citrus peel

Directions

1. Combine all the ingredients and mix well.

2. Store in a spray bottle.

Citrus Surface Cleaner

Choose this homemade recipe to keep your house clean

Ingredients

1 cup distilled vinegar

1 cup water

½ lemon, juiced

10 drops Sweet Orange essential oil

Directions

1. Mix all the ingredients.

2. Store in a spray bottle

Safe Surface Cleaner

<u>Ingredients</u>

8 drops Mandarin essential oil

1 cup water

<u>Directions</u>

Combine to a spray bottle.

Use to wipe down surfaces in baby's room.